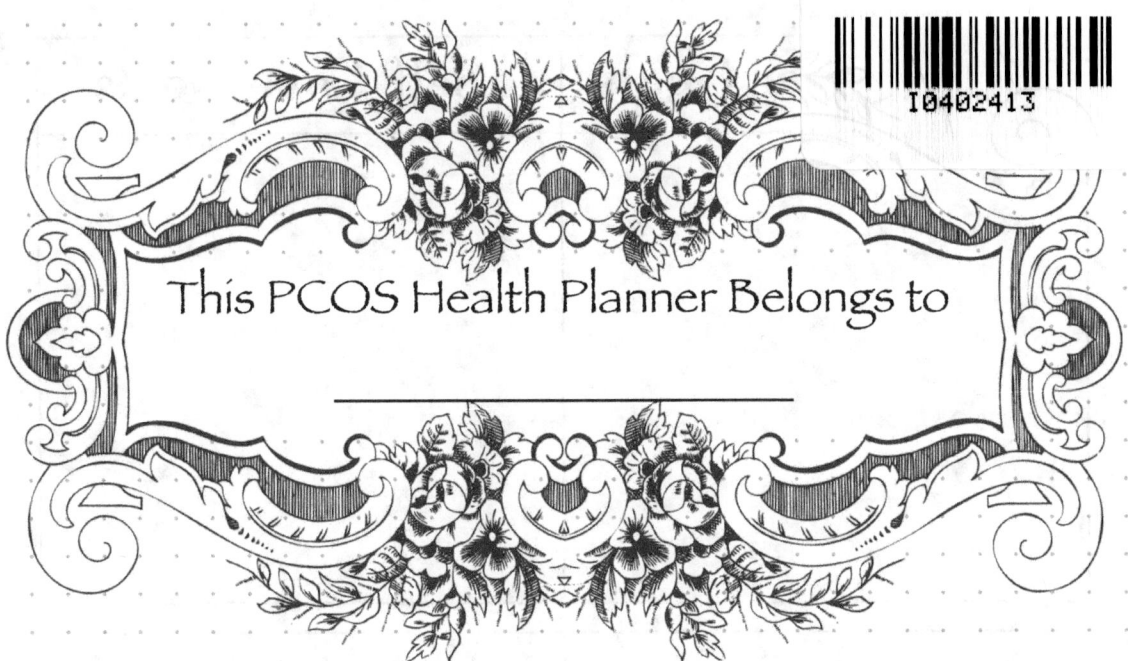

This PCOS Health Planner Belongs to

_____

New Career Goals	Self-Love Goals

Exercise Goals	New Activity Goals

Trip Planning Goals	Self-Care Goals

January Events	February Events

April Events	March Events

May Events	June Events

Summer Goals	Travel Goals

New Mindset Goals	Fall Activity Goals

Holiday Goals	New Year Goals

July Events	August Events

September Events	October Events

November Events	December Events

Introduction

- **What exactly is PCOS ?** Polycystic ovary syndrome is a commonly known hormonal disorder that effects women who are of the age of reproduction. It can start in young girls at as early of the age of 11 and effect women all the way up to the age of 50. But the most common cases occur between the age of 18-45.

- **Although the exact cause of PCOS is not known -** If you are experiencing symptoms like: severe breakouts of acne, excess body or facial hair, male pattern baldness (thinning on the top or front of your head), infrequent or irregular menstrual cycles, weight issues due to hormonal imbalances, unexplained hypertension, skin discoloration, increased feelings of anxiety or stress, bouts of depression or if PCOS runs in your family. I would recommend seeing your Doctor. Once diagnosed there are things that you can start doing on your own to help reduce the risk of experiencing any long term complications in the future.

- **Adapt a Regular Consumption/Eating Schedule -** Eating at regularly scheduled intervals will program your body to better process foods after surgery. It will also help to regulate your hormones, reduce body weight, stabilize blood sugar & cholesterol levels, & regulate sleeping patterns.

- **Adapt a Regular Exercise Schedule -** The best time to Exercise is whenever you can. But by adapting a schedule it will make it easier to adjust. For most people the best time if possible to exercise is in the mornings, because you will rarely have things that interfere with your schedule. Exercise also increases your productivity & mental clarity, releases endorphins and sparks your metabolism, helps reduce stress & promotes healthier skin. Another benefit of morning exercise is, it gets your workout done so that you can focus on other things throughout the day.

More Information

- **Genetics/Heredity -** Studies show that certain Genes may be linked to PCOS. For instance insulin resistance from either side of the family can be passed down & can be an attributing cause, and although some women don't experience symptoms until their late 20's or early 30's, studies show that if you have PCOS you were born with it.

- **Physical Changes & Problems-** For the most part the problem is that your body is producing too much androgen. This is why it is harder for you to become pregnant, and why you are growing excess hair, and if not treated PCOS can lead to more serious (if those weren't serious enough) problems like heart disease & even cancer. Another effect of PCOS are the cyst that basically attack your ovaries, these can lead to major hormonal imbalances. But wait it gets worse! PCOS also increases your risk for strokes & can possibly lead to death...

- **Complications -** There are also other complications that are associated with PCOS which include:
    - Abnormal Uterine Bleeding
    - Endometrial Cancer (Cancer of your Uterine lining)
    - Gestational Diabetes (aka Pregnancy induced ↑BP)
    - Infertility
    - Metabolic Syndrome
    - Miscarriage or Premature Births
    - Nonalcoholic Steatohepatitis (A fatty liver disease)
    - Obesity can also complicate PCOS by exacerbating the metabolic, psychological & reproductive features of the disease.

Treatment

- **Lifestyle Changes -** Although your Doctor may prescribe you medications, to regulate your menstrual cycle, help you ovulate, or reduce hair growth. Be aware that with every new thing that you put into your body, there will come more side effects & symptoms to deal with. So for the most part you need to adapt a healthy lifestyle, so that you can stimulate normal processes on your own, and be able to deal with the added stress from the medications.

- **Avoid Negative Stress -** Avoid negative people, negative self-talk and negative thinking. Negative thinking triggers hormones in our bodies that can lead to bouts of anxiety, depression & mood disorders. It's important to get in at least 30 minutes of exercise every day to help your body & mind detox & release stress through that avenue. Exercise will also help lower your blood sugar levels, help prevent insulin resistance and help you to manage your weight. I recommend meeting with a professional that can help you put together a resistance/weight program and a complimenting cardio program as well.

- **Journal -** Utilize your journal in the back to vent & release your thoughts & emotions when needed. Journaling will also help you reach your goals, strengthen your self-discipline & increase self-confidence. The last thing that you want to do, is let your emotions pile up.

- **Cookbook -** Utilize your cookbook to log meals that are healthy & that give you good energy throughout the day. Most Doctors recommend Low Carb Meals. But I would say, opt for more complex carbs & whole grains. But overall we all metabolize foods differently. So the key is to write down how you feel approximately 1 hour after eating this will give you the best feedback in regards to what you should or shouldn't be eating. If you feel like you have enough energy for another hour or two, I would say that is a good meal for you, so log in your recipe book. If not, try adding a little more healthy fats, or protein. But not both at the same time.

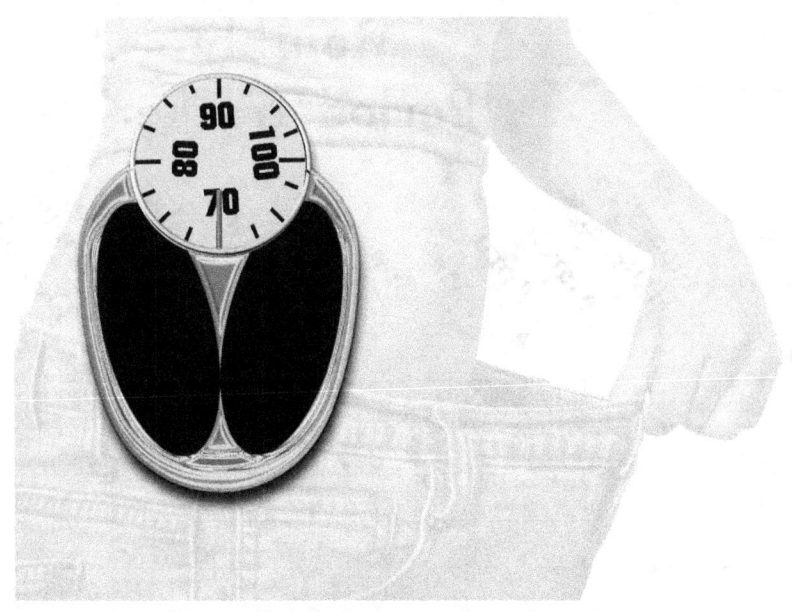

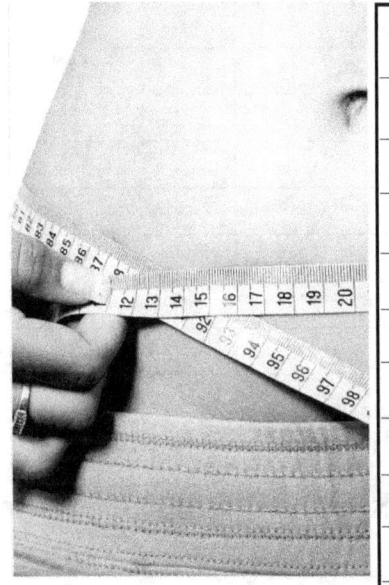

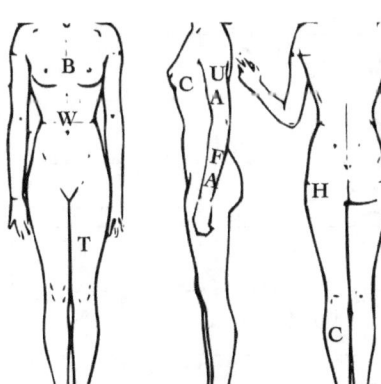

Measurements

Weight		Body Mass Index (BMI)	
Body Fat %		Water Weight	
Bust		Muscle Weight	
Chest		**Ok How are we Looking?**	
Waist			
Hips			
Thighs			
Calves			
Upper Arm			
Fore Arm			

How do you feel Overall about your measurements?

How do you feel Overall?

What do you think will be your biggest challenge?

What can you do to overcome that challenge?

Monthly Period Tracker

Cycle Day	January	February	March	April	May	June	July	August	September	October	November	December	Mode	Normal/Cool	Heavy/Stress
1															
2															☂
3															
4															
5															
6															💧
7															
8															💧
9															
10															
11															🎭
12															⚡
13															
14															😞

Cycle

Sprinkle   **Light**   **Medium**   **Heavy**

Notes/Comments

Vacations
Important Dates

_____   _____
_____   _____
_____   _____
_____   _____
_____   _____
_____   _____
_____   _____

Monthly Ovulation Tracker

Cycle Day	January	February	March	April	May	June	July	August	September	October	November	December	Mode	Period Started/P	Ovulation/OT
1														p	
2															
3															
4															
5															
6															
7															
8															
9															
10															
11															ot
12															ot
13															ot
14															ot
15															ot
16															ot
17															ot
18															
19															
20															
21															
22															
23															
24															
25															
26															
27															
28															
29															
30															
31															

30 Day Misc. Habit Tracker

Day						Smoking								
1						X								
2						X								
3						X								
4						X								
5						X								
6						X								
7						X								
8						X								
9						X								
10						X								
11														
12														
13														
14														
15														
16														
17														
18														
19														
20														
21														
22														
23														
24														
25														
26														
27														
28														
29														
30														
31														

30 Day Misc. Habit Tracker

Day						Snacks							
1						x							
2						x							
3						x							
4						x							
5						x							
6						x							
7						x							
8						x							
9						x							
10						x							
11													
12													
13													
14													
15													
16													
17													
18													
19													
20													
21													
22													
23													
24													
25													
26													
27													
28													
29													
30													
31													

30 Day Misc. Habit Tracker

Day						Shopping									
1															
2															
3															
4															
5															
6															
7															
8															
9															
10															
11															
12															
13															
14															
15															
16															
17															
18															
19															
20															
21															
22															
23															
24															
25															
26															
27															
28															
29															
30															
31															

January 2020

Sun	Mon	Tue	Wed	Thu	Fri	Sat
Feelings Events Dates	Notes Appoint. Birthdays	31	1	2	3	4
5	6	7	8	9	10	11
12	13	14	15	16	17	18
19	20 MLK	21	22	23	24	25
26	27	28	29	30	31	1

Monthly Overview/Notes
_____
_____
_____

Put a check mark if you ate on time!	Brkfast	Lunch	Dinner
Monday	🎭		
Tuesday	✓		
Wednesday			
Thursday			
Friday			
Saturday			
Sunday			

🎭 1 hr After each meal write an emoji for how you feel as far as energy, happy for good sad for bad!

Habit Tracker

Positive Pick New	Negative Pick Old
T	
W	F

Use The initials of each day to track Your New & Old Habits

Water Intake	64oz. 's
Monday	
Tuesday	
Wednesday	
Thursday	
Friday	
Saturday	
Sunday	

Weekly Menu

Monday:

Tuesday:

Wednesday:

Thursday:

Friday:

Weekend:

Saturday	Sunday

Exercise/ Cardio 🏃	🕐
Monday	
Tuesday	
Wednesday	
Thursday	
Friday	
Saturday	
Sunday	

Specify whether Cardio or Strength Training. E/C

Put a check mark if you ate on time!	Brkfast	Lunch	Dinner
Monday	🎭		
Tuesday	✓		
Wednesday			
Thursday			
Friday			
Saturday			
Sunday			

🎭 1 hr After each meal write an emoji for how you feel as far as energy, happy for good sad for bad!

Habit Tracker

Positive Pick New	Negative Pick Old
T	
W	F

Use The initials of each day to track Your New & Old Habits

Water Intake	64oz. 's
Monday	
Tuesday	
Wednesday	
Thursday	
Friday	
Saturday	
Sunday	

Weekly Menu

Monday:

Tuesday:

Wednesday:

Thursday:

Friday:

Weekend:

Saturday	Sunday

Exercise/ Cardio		
Monday		
Tuesday		
Wednesday		
Thursday		
Friday		
Saturday		
Sunday		

Specify whether Cardio or Strength Training. E/C

Put a check mark if you ate on time!	Brkfast	Lunch	Dinner
Monday	🎭		
Tuesday	✓		
Wednesday			
Thursday			
Friday			
Saturday			
Sunday			

🎭 1 hr After each meal write an emoji for how you feel as far as energy, happy for good sad for bad!

Habit Tracker

Positive Pick New	Negative Pick Old
T	
W	F

Use The initials of each day to track Your New & Old Habits

Water Intake	64oz 🥛's
Monday	
Tuesday	
Wednesday	
Thursday	
Friday	
Saturday	
Sunday	

Weekly Menu

Monday:

Tuesday:

Wednesday:

Thursday:

Friday:

Weekend:

Saturday	Sunday

Exercise/ Cardio 🏋️🚶 🕐	
Monday	
Tuesday	
Wednesday	
Thursday	
Friday	
Saturday	
Sunday	

Specify whether Cardio or Strength Training. E/C

Put a check mark if you ate on time!	Brkfast	Lunch	Dinner
Monday	🎭		
Tuesday	✓		
Wednesday			
Thursday			
Friday			
Saturday			
Sunday			

🎭 1 hr After each meal write an emoji for how you feel as far as energy, happy for good sad for bad!

Habit Tracker

Positive Pick New	Negative Pick Old
T	
W	F

Use The initials of each day to track Your New & Old Habits

Water Intake	64oz. 's
Monday	
Tuesday	
Wednesday	
Thursday	
Friday	
Saturday	
Sunday	

Exercise/ Cardio 🏋️ 🕒	
Monday	
Tuesday	
Wednesday	
Thursday	
Friday	
Saturday	
Sunday	

Specify whether Cardio or Strength Training. E/C

Weekly Menu

Monday:

Tuesday:

Wednesday:

Thursday:

Friday:

Weekend:

Saturday	Sunday

February 2020

Sun	Mon	Tue	Wed	Thu	Fri	Sat
Things To-Do List Or Remember 1. 2.		28	29	30	31	. 1
2	3	4 **RosaParks**	5	6	7	8
9	10	11	12 **Lin.Bday**	13	14 ♥	15 **Susan B.**
16	17 **Was.Bday**	18	19	20	21	22
23	24	25	26 **Ash**	27	28	29

Monthly Overview/Notes

_____
_____
_____

Put a check mark if you ate on time!	Brkfast	Lunch	Dinner
Monday	🎭		
Tuesday	✓		
Wednesday			
Thursday			
Friday			
Saturday			
Sunday			

🎭 1 hr After each meal write an emoji for how you feel as far as energy, happy for good sad for bad!

Habit Tracker

Positive Pick New	Negative Pick Old
T	
W	F

Use The initials of each day to track Your New & Old Habits

Water Intake	64oz 🥤 's
Monday	
Tuesday	
Wednesday	
Thursday	
Friday	
Saturday	
Sunday	

Exercise/ Cardio 🏋️🏃 🕐	
Monday	
Tuesday	
Wednesday	
Thursday	
Friday	
Saturday	
Sunday	

Specify whether Cardio or Strength Training. E/C

Weekly Menu

Monday:

Tuesday:

Wednesday:

Thursday:

Friday:

Weekend:

Saturday	Sunday

What are some New foods you can try make a list?	Brkfast	Lunch	Dinner
Monday			
Tuesday			
Wednesday			
Thursday			
Friday			
Saturday			
Sunday			

1 hr After each meal mark how you feel as far as energy, with the New Foods from Your list !

New Habits

What are some New things that You would like to try?
1.
2.
3.

Okay Pick one & Track

M	T	W	Th	F	S	S

Put a check mark each day to track Your New Habit for the next 6 Weeks

Water Intake	64oz.'s
Week 1	
Week 2	
Week 3	
Week 4	
Week 5	

Has drinking the 64oz.'s been an issue? Are you sipping regularly throughout the day?

Exercise/ Cardio	E	C
Week 1		
Week 2		
Week 3		
Week 4		
Week 5		

Fill in how many hours You Trained for each week

Progress Assessment

1-10 How do I feel about my progress/surgery?

How many pounds have I lost?

How do I look in the mirror?

Do I like what I see so far?

What has been the hardest adjustment/s thus far?

What can I do to make this transition easier?

Who can I call or count on for support?

Put a check mark if you ate on time!	Brkfast	Lunch	Dinner
Monday	🎭		
Tuesday	✓		
Wednesday			
Thursday			
Friday			
Saturday			
Sunday			

🎭🎭 1 hr After each meal write an emoji for how you feel as far as energy, happy for good sad for bad!

Habit Tracker

Positive Pick New	Negative Pick Old
T	
W	F

Use The initials of each day to track Your New & Old Habits

Water Intake	64oz. 's
Monday	
Tuesday	
Wednesday	
Thursday	
Friday	
Saturday	
Sunday	

Exercise/ Cardio 🏋️🚶🕐	
Monday	
Tuesday	
Wednesday	
Thursday	
Friday	
Saturday	
Sunday	

Specify whether Cardio or Strength Training. E/C

Weekly Menu

Monday:

Tuesday:

Wednesday:

Thursday:

Friday:

Weekend:

Saturday	Sunday

Put a check mark if you ate on time!	Brkfast	Lunch	Dinner
Monday	🎭		
Tuesday	✓		
Wednesday			
Thursday			
Friday			
Saturday			
Sunday			

🎭 1 hr After each meal write an emoji for how you feel as far as energy, happy for good sad for bad!

Habit Tracker	
Positive	Negative
Pick New	Pick Old
T	
W	F

Use The initials of each day to track Your New & Old Habits

Water Intake	64oz. 's
Monday	
Tuesday	
Wednesday	
Thursday	
Friday	
Saturday	
Sunday	

Weekly Menu

Monday:

Tuesday:

Wednesday:

Thursday:

Friday:

Weekend:

Saturday	Sunday

Exercise/ 🏋 Cardio 🏃	🕒
Monday	
Tuesday	
Wednesday	
Thursday	
Friday	
Saturday	
Sunday	

Specify whether Cardio or Strength Training. E/C

Put a check mark if you ate on time!	Brkfast	Lunch	Dinner
Monday	🎭		
Tuesday	✓		
Wednesday			
Thursday			
Friday			
Saturday			
Sunday			

🎭 1 hr After each meal write an emoji for how you feel as far as energy, happy for good sad for bad!

Habit Tracker

Positive Pick New	Negative Pick Old
T	
W	F

Use The initials of each day to track Your New & Old Habits

Water Intake	64oz. 's
Monday	
Tuesday	
Wednesday	
Thursday	
Friday	
Saturday	
Sunday	

Weekly Menu

Monday:

Tuesday:

Wednesday:

Thursday:

Friday:

Weekend:

Saturday	Sunday

Exercise/ Cardio 🏋️ 🏃 🕒	
Monday	
Tuesday	
Wednesday	
Thursday	
Friday	
Saturday	
Sunday	

Specify whether Cardio or Strength Training. E/C

March 2020

Sun	Mon	Tue	Wed	Thu	Fri	Sat
1	2	3	4	5	6	7
8	9	10 **Purim**	11	12	13	14
15	16	17 **St. Pat's**	18	19 **Equinox**	20	21
22	23	24	25	26	27	28
29	30	31	1	2	3	

Monthly Overview/Notes

Put a check mark if you ate on time!	Brkfast	Lunch	Dinner
Monday	🎭		
Tuesday	✓		
Wednesday			
Thursday			
Friday			
Saturday			
Sunday			

🎭 1 hr After each meal write an emoji for how you feel as far as energy, happy for good sad for bad!

Habit Tracker

Positive Pick New	Negative Pick Old
T	
W	F

Use The initials of each day to track Your New & Old Habits

Water Intake	64oz 's
Monday	
Tuesday	
Wednesday	
Thursday	
Friday	
Saturday	
Sunday	

Exercise/ Cardio		
Monday		
Tuesday		
Wednesday		
Thursday		
Friday		
Saturday		
Sunday		

Specify whether Cardio or Strength Training. E/C

Weekly Menu

Monday:

Tuesday:

Wednesday:

Thursday:

Friday:

Weekend:

Saturday	Sunday

Put a check mark if you ate on time!	Brkfast	Lunch	Dinner
Monday	🎭		
Tuesday	✓		
Wednesday			
Thursday			
Friday			
Saturday			
Sunday			

🎭 1 hr After each meal write an emoji for how you feel as far as energy, happy for good sad for bad!

Habit Tracker

Positive Pick New	Negative Pick Old
T	
W	F

Use The initials of each day to track Your New & Old Habits

Water Intake	64oz. 's
Monday	
Tuesday	
Wednesday	
Thursday	
Friday	
Saturday	
Sunday	

Exercise/ Cardio 🏋🏃 🕐	
Monday	
Tuesday	
Wednesday	
Thursday	
Friday	
Saturday	
Sunday	

Specify whether Cardio or Strength Training. E/C

Weekly Menu

Monday:

Tuesday:

Wednesday:

Thursday:

Friday:

Weekend:

Saturday	Sunday

What are some New foods you can try make a list?	Brkfast	Lunch	Dinner
Monday			
Tuesday			
Wednesday			
Thursday			
Friday			
Saturday			
Sunday			

1 hr After each meal mark how you feel as far as energy, with the New Foods from Your list!

New Habits

What are some New things that You would like to try?
1. _____
2. _____
3. _____

Okay Pick one & Track

M	T	W	Th	F	S	S

Put a check mark each day to track Your New Habit for the next 6 Weeks

Water Intake	64oz. 's
Week 11	
Week 12	
Week 13	
Week 14	
Week 15	

Fill in how many 12oz. cups You drank each week

Exercise/Cardio	E	C
Week 11		
Week 12		
Week 13		
Week 14		
Week 15		

Fill in how many hours You Trained for each week

Progress Assessment

1-10 How do I feel about my progress?

How many pounds have I lost?

How many inches have I lost?

How do I look in the mirror?

What size is my clothing now?

Have I bought new clothes yet?

How has my energy been lately?

How have my workouts been?

Is it easier to plan my meals?

Have I received any compliments lately?

What do I like most, the way I feel or look?

What is a new food/recipe that I've tried lately?

Have I met any new friends or likeminded people?

How has the journey been thus far?

Put a check mark if you ate on time!	Brkfast	Lunch	Dinner
Monday	🎭		
Tuesday	✓		
Wednesday			
Thursday			
Friday			
Saturday			
Sunday			

🎭 1 hr After each meal write an emoji for how you feel as far as energy, happy for good sad for bad!

Habit Tracker

Positive Pick New	Negative Pick Old
T	
W	F

Use The initials of each day to track Your New & Old Habits

Water Intake	64oz. 🥛's
Monday	
Tuesday	
Wednesday	
Thursday	
Friday	
Saturday	
Sunday	

Weekly Menu

Monday:

Tuesday:

Wednesday:

Thursday:

Friday:

Weekend:

Saturday	Sunday

Exercise/ Cardio 🏋️🏃🕐	
Monday	
Tuesday	
Wednesday	
Thursday	
Friday	
Saturday	
Sunday	

Specify whether Cardio or Strength Training. E/C

Put a check mark if you ate on time!	Brkfast	Lunch	Dinner
Monday	🎭		
Tuesday	✓		
Wednesday			
Thursday			
Friday			
Saturday			
Sunday			

🎭 1 hr After each meal write an emoji for how you feel as far as energy, happy for good sad for bad!

Habit Tracker

Positive Pick New	Negative Pick Old
T	
W	F

Use The initials of each day to track Your New & Old Habits

Water Intake	64oz. 's
Monday	
Tuesday	
Wednesday	
Thursday	
Friday	
Saturday	
Sunday	

Exercise/ Cardio 🏋🚶	🕐
Monday	
Tuesday	
Wednesday	
Thursday	
Friday	
Saturday	
Sunday	

Specify whether Cardio or Strength Training. E/C

Weekly Menu

Monday:

Tuesday:

Wednesday:

Thursday:

Friday:

Weekend:

Saturday	Sunday

Put a check mark if you ate on time!	Brkfast	Lunch	Dinner		
Monday	🎭				
Tuesday	✓				
Wednesday					
Thursday					
Friday					
Saturday					
Sunday					

🎭 1 hr After each meal write an emoji for how you feel as far as energy, happy for good sad for bad!

Habit Tracker

Positive Pick New	Negative Pick Old
T	
W	F

Use The initials of each day to track Your New & Old Habits

Water Intake	64oz. 's
Monday	
Tuesday	
Wednesday	
Thursday	
Friday	
Saturday	
Sunday	

Weekly Menu

Monday:

Tuesday:

Wednesday:

Thursday:

Friday:

Weekend:

Saturday	Sunday

Exercise/ Cardio 🏋️ 🏃	🕐
Monday	
Tuesday	
Wednesday	
Thursday	
Friday	
Saturday	
Sunday	

Specify whether Cardio or Strength Training. E/C

April 2020

Sun	Mon	Tue	Wed	Thu	Fri	Sat
	30	31	1	2	3	4
5 Palm	6	7	8	9 PassOver	10 Good	11
12 Easter	13	14	15 TaxDay	16 LD/PasOv	17	18
19	20	21 Yom HaS.	22	23	24 Ramadan	25
26	27	28	29 Yom Ha'a	30	1	2

Monthly Overview/Notes

_____
_____
_____
_____

Put a check mark if you ate on time!	Brkfast	Lunch	Dinner
Monday			
Tuesday	✓		
Wednesday			
Thursday			
Friday			
Saturday			
Sunday			

🎭 1 hr After each meal write an emoji for how you feel as far as energy, happy for good sad for bad!

Habit Tracker

Positive Pick New		Negative Pick Old	
T			
W			F

Use The initials of each day to track Your New & Old Habits

Water Intake	64oz. 🥛's
Monday	
Tuesday	
Wednesday	
Thursday	
Friday	
Saturday	
Sunday	

Exercise/ Cardio 🏋️🏃 🕐	
Monday	
Tuesday	
Wednesday	
Thursday	
Friday	
Saturday	
Sunday	

Specify whether Cardio or Strength Training. E/C

Weekly Menu

Monday:

Tuesday:

Wednesday:

Thursday:

Friday:

Weekend:

Saturday	Sunday

Put a check mark if you ate on time!	Brkfast	Lunch	Dinner
Monday	🎭		
Tuesday	✓		
Wednesday			
Thursday			
Friday			
Saturday			
Sunday			

🎭 1 hr After each meal write an emoji for how you feel as far as energy, happy for good sad for bad!

Habit Tracker

Positive Pick New	Negative Pick Old
T	
W	F

Use The initials of each day to track Your New & Old Habits

Water Intake	64oz. 🥛's
Monday	
Tuesday	
Wednesday	
Thursday	
Friday	
Saturday	
Sunday	

Exercise/ Cardio 🏋️ 🚶 🕒	
Monday	
Tuesday	
Wednesday	
Thursday	
Friday	
Saturday	
Sunday	

Specify whether Cardio or Strength Training. E/C

Weekly Menu

Monday:

Tuesday:

Wednesday:

Thursday:

Friday:

Weekend:

Saturday   Sunday

Put a check mark if you ate on time!	Brkfast	Lunch	Dinner
Monday	🎭		
Tuesday	✓		
Wednesday			
Thursday			
Friday			
Saturday			
Sunday			

🎭 1 hr After each meal write an emoji for how you feel as far as energy, happy for good sad for bad!

Habit Tracker

Positive Pick New	Negative Pick Old
T	
W	F

Use The initials of each day to track Your New & Old Habits

Water Intake	64oz. 's
Monday	
Tuesday	
Wednesday	
Thursday	
Friday	
Saturday	
Sunday	

Weekly Menu

Monday:

Tuesday:

Wednesday:

Thursday:

Friday:

Weekend:

Saturday	Sunday

Exercise/ Cardio 🏋🏃	🕐
Monday	
Tuesday	
Wednesday	
Thursday	
Friday	
Saturday	
Sunday	

Specify whether Cardio or Strength Training. E/C

Put a check mark if you ate on time!	Brkfast	Lunch	Dinner
Monday	🎭		
Tuesday	✓		
Wednesday			
Thursday			
Friday			
Saturday			
Sunday			

🎭 1 hr After each meal write an emoji for how you feel as far as energy, happy for good sad for bad!

Habit Tracker

Positive Pick New	Negative Pick Old
T	
W	F

Use The initials of each day to track Your New & Old Habits

Water Intake	64oz. 's	
Monday		
Tuesday		
Wednesday		
Thursday		
Friday		
Saturday		
Sunday		

Exercise/ Cardio 🏃		
Monday		
Tuesday		
Wednesday		
Thursday		
Friday		
Saturday		
Sunday		

Specify whether Cardio or Strength Training. E/C

Weekly Menu

Monday:

Tuesday:

Wednesday:

Thursday:

Friday:

Weekend:

Saturday	Sunday

Put a check mark if you ate on time!	Brkfast	Lunch	Dinner
Monday	🎭		
Tuesday	✓		
Wednesday			
Thursday			
Friday			
Saturday			
Sunday			

🎭 1 hr After each meal write an emoji for how you feel as far as energy, happy for good sad for bad!

Habit Tracker

Positive Pick New		Negative Pick Old	
	T		
W			F

Use The initials of each day to track Your New & Old Habits

Water Intake	64oz. 's
Monday	
Tuesday	
Wednesday	
Thursday	
Friday	
Saturday	
Sunday	

Exercise/ Cardio 🏋️🚶 🕐	
Monday	
Tuesday	
Wednesday	
Thursday	
Friday	
Saturday	
Sunday	

Specify whether Cardio or Strength Training. E/C

Weekly Menu

Monday:

Tuesday:

Wednesday:

Thursday:

Friday:

Weekend:

Saturday	Sunday

May 2020

Sun	Mon	Tue	Wed	Thu	Fri	Sat
	27	28	29	30	1	2
3	4	5 Cinco de	6	7	8	9
10 Mother's	11	12 Lag BaO	13	14	15	16
17	18	19	20	21	22	23
24	25 Memorial	26	27	28	29 Shavuot	30
31	1	2	3	4	5	6

Monthly Overview/Notes

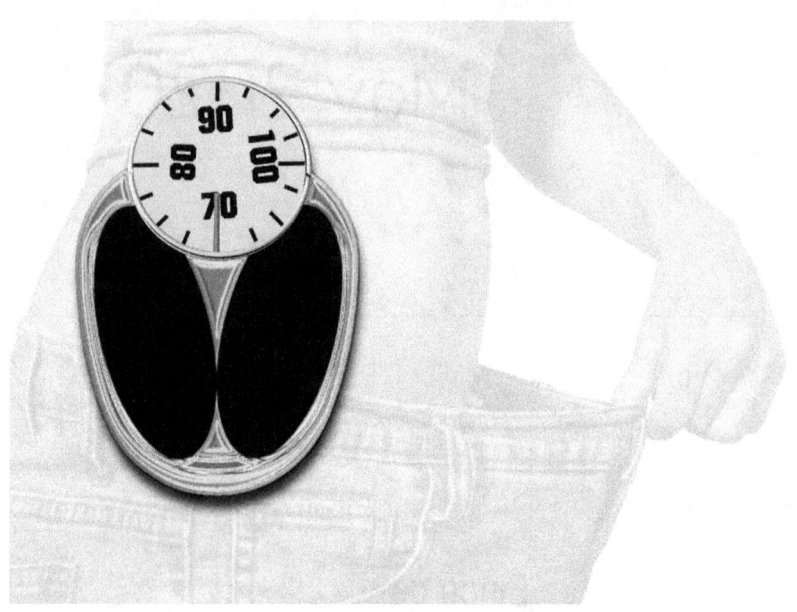

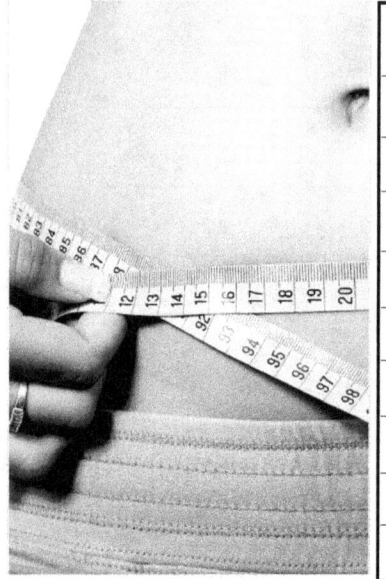

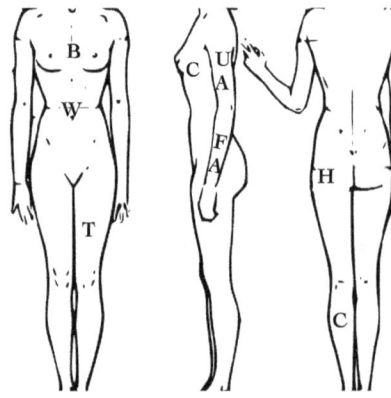

Measurements			
Weight		Body Mass Index (BMI)	
Body Fat %		Water Weight	
Bust		Muscle Weight	
Chest		**Notes**	
Waist			
Hips			
Thighs			
Calves			
Upper Arm			
Fore Arm			

Well how is it going?????

How do you feel Overall?

Are you happy with your progress so far?

What have you cut out? Are you seeing more results?

Put a check mark if you ate on time!	Brkfast	Lunch	Dinner
Monday	🎭		
Tuesday	✓		
Wednesday			
Thursday			
Friday			
Saturday			
Sunday			

🎭 1 hr After each meal write an emoji for how you feel as far as energy, happy for good sad for bad!

Habit Tracker

Positive Pick New	Negative Pick Old
T	
W	F

Use The initials of each day to track Your New & Old Habits

Water Intake	64oz. 's
Monday	
Tuesday	
Wednesday	
Thursday	
Friday	
Saturday	
Sunday	

Weekly Menu

Monday:

Tuesday:

Wednesday:

Thursday:

Friday:

Weekend:

Saturday	Sunday

Exercise/Cardio		
Monday		
Tuesday		
Wednesday		
Thursday		
Friday		
Saturday		
Sunday		

Specify whether Cardio or Strength Training. E/C

Put a check mark if you ate on time!	Brkfast	Lunch	Dinner
Monday	😷		
Tuesday	✓		
Wednesday			
Thursday			
Friday			
Saturday			
Sunday			

🎭 1 hr After each meal write an emoji for how you feel as far as energy, happy for good sad for bad!

Habit Tracker

Positive Pick New	Negative Pick Old
T	
W	F

Use The initials of each day to track Your New & Old Habits

Water Intake	64oz. 🥛's
Monday	
Tuesday	
Wednesday	
Thursday	
Friday	
Saturday	
Sunday	

Exercise/ Cardio 🏋🚶 🕐	
Monday	
Tuesday	
Wednesday	
Thursday	
Friday	
Saturday	
Sunday	

Specify whether Cardio or Strength Training. E/C

Weekly Menu

Monday:

Tuesday:

Wednesday:

Thursday:

Friday:

Weekend:

Saturday	Sunday

Put a check mark if you ate on time!	Brkfast	Lunch	Dinner
Monday	🎭		
Tuesday	✓		
Wednesday			
Thursday			
Friday			
Saturday			
Sunday			

1 hr After each meal write an emoji for how you feel as far as energy, happy for good sad for bad!

Habit Tracker

Positive Pick New	Negative Pick Old
T	
W	F

Use The initials of each day to track Your New & Old Habits

Water Intake	64oz. 's
Monday	
Tuesday	
Wednesday	
Thursday	
Friday	
Saturday	
Sunday	

Exercise/ Cardio	
Monday	
Tuesday	
Wednesday	
Thursday	
Friday	
Saturday	
Sunday	

Specify whether Cardio or Strength Training. E/C

Weekly Menu

Monday:

Tuesday:

Wednesday:

Thursday:

Friday:

Weekend:

Saturday	Sunday

Put a check mark if you ate on time!	Brkfast	Lunch	Dinner
Monday	🎭		
Tuesday	✓		
Wednesday			
Thursday			
Friday			
Saturday			
Sunday			

🎭 1 hr After each meal write an emoji for how you feel as far as energy, happy for good sad for bad!

Habit Tracker

Positive Pick New	Negative Pick Old
T	
W	F

Use The initials of each day to track Your New & Old Habits

Water Intake	64oz. 's
Monday	
Tuesday	
Wednesday	
Thursday	
Friday	
Saturday	
Sunday	

Exercise/ Cardio 🏋🏃 🕒	
Monday	
Tuesday	
Wednesday	
Thursday	
Friday	
Saturday	
Sunday	

Specify whether Cardio or Strength Training. E/C

Weekly Menu

Monday:

Tuesday:

Wednesday:

Thursday:

Friday:

Weekend:

Saturday	Sunday

Put a check mark if you ate on time!	Brkfast	Lunch	Dinner
Monday	🎭		
Tuesday	✓		
Wednesday			
Thursday			
Friday			
Saturday			
Sunday			

🎭 1 hr After each meal write an emoji for how you feel as far as energy, happy for good sad for bad!

Habit Tracker

Positive Pick New	Negative Pick Old
T	
W	F

Use The initials of each day to track Your New & Old Habits

Water Intake	64oz. 's
Monday	
Tuesday	
Wednesday	
Thursday	
Friday	
Saturday	
Sunday	

Weekly Menu

Monday:

Tuesday:

Wednesday:

Thursday:

Friday:

Weekend:

Saturday	Sunday

Exercise/ Cardio 🏃 🏋️ 🕐	
Monday	
Tuesday	
Wednesday	
Thursday	
Friday	
Saturday	
Sunday	

Specify whether Cardio or Strength Training. E/C

June 2020

Sun	Mon	Tue	Wed	Thu	Fri	Sat
	1	2	3	4	5	6
7	8	9	10	11	12	13
14 Army	15	16	17	18	19 Teenth	20 Solstice
21 Father's	22	23	24	25	26	27
28	29	30	1	2	3	4

Monthly Overview/Notes

_____
_____
_____
_____

Put a check mark if you ate on time!	Brkfast	Lunch	Dinner
Monday	🎭		
Tuesday	✓		
Wednesday			
Thursday			
Friday			
Saturday			
Sunday			

🎭 1 hr After each meal write an emoji for how you feel as far as energy, happy for good sad for bad!

Habit Tracker

Positive Pick New	Negative Pick Old
T	
W	F

Use The initials of each day to track Your New & Old Habits

Water Intake	64oz.'s
Monday	
Tuesday	
Wednesday	
Thursday	
Friday	
Saturday	
Sunday	

Weekly Menu

Monday:
_____
_____

Tuesday:
_____
_____

Wednesday:
_____
_____

Thursday:
_____
_____

Friday:
_____
_____

Weekend:

Saturday	Sunday

Exercise/ Cardio 🏋️🚶	🕐
Monday	
Tuesday	
Wednesday	
Thursday	
Friday	
Saturday	
Sunday	

Specify whether Cardio or Strength Training. E/C

Put a check mark if you ate on time!	Brkfast	Lunch	Dinner
Monday	🎭		
Tuesday	✓		
Wednesday			
Thursday			
Friday			
Saturday			
Sunday			

🎭 1 hr After each meal write an emoji for how you feel as far as energy, happy for good sad for bad!

Habit Tracker

Positive Pick New	Negative Pick Old
T	
W	F

Use The initials of each day to track Your New & Old Habits

Water Intake	64oz. 's
Monday	
Tuesday	
Wednesday	
Thursday	
Friday	
Saturday	
Sunday	

Exercise/Cardio 🏋️ 🏃 🕒	
Monday	
Tuesday	
Wednesday	
Thursday	
Friday	
Saturday	
Sunday	

Specify whether Cardio or Strength Training. E/C

Weekly Menu

Monday:

Tuesday:

Wednesday:

Thursday:

Friday:

Weekend:

Saturday	Sunday

Put a check mark if you ate on time!	Brkfast	Lunch	Dinner
Monday	🎭		
Tuesday	✓		
Wednesday			
Thursday			
Friday			
Saturday			
Sunday			

🎭 1 hr After each meal write an emoji for how you feel as far as energy, happy for good sad for bad!

Habit Tracker

Positive Pick New	Negative Pick Old
T	
W	F

Use The initials of each day to track Your New & Old Habits

Water Intake	64oz. 🥛's
Monday	
Tuesday	
Wednesday	
Thursday	
Friday	
Saturday	
Sunday	

Exercise/Cardio 🏋️🚶🕐	
Monday	
Tuesday	
Wednesday	
Thursday	
Friday	
Saturday	
Sunday	

Specify whether Cardio or Strength Training. E/C

Weekly Menu

Monday:

Tuesday:

Wednesday:

Thursday:

Friday:

Weekend:

Saturday | Sunday

Put a check mark if you ate on time!	Brkfast	Lunch	Dinner
Monday			
Tuesday	✓		
Wednesday			
Thursday			
Friday			
Saturday			
Sunday			

1 hr After each meal write an emoji for how you feel as far as energy, happy for good sad for bad!

Habit Tracker

Positive Pick New	Negative Pick Old
T	
W	F

Use The initials of each day to track Your New & Old Habits

Water Intake	64oz. 's
Monday	
Tuesday	
Wednesday	
Thursday	
Friday	
Saturday	
Sunday	

Exercise/ Cardio	
Monday	
Tuesday	
Wednesday	
Thursday	
Friday	
Saturday	
Sunday	

Specify whether Cardio or Strength Training. E/C

Weekly Menu

Monday:

Tuesday:

Wednesday:

Thursday:

Friday:

Weekend:

Saturday	Sunday

July 2020

Sun	Mon	Tue	Wed	Thu	Fri	Sat
	29	30	1	2	3	4 **Indepen.**
5	6	7	8	9	10	11
12	13	14	15	16	17	18
19	20	21	22	23	24	25
26	27	28	29	30 **TishaB'Av**	31	1

Monthly Overview/Notes

_____
_____
_____
_____

Put a check mark if you ate on time!	Brkfast	Lunch	Dinner
Monday	🎭		
Tuesday	✓		
Wednesday			
Thursday			
Friday			
Saturday			
Sunday			

🎭 1 hr After each meal write an emoji for how you feel as far as energy, happy for good sad for bad!

Habit Tracker

Positive Pick New	Negative Pick Old
T	
W	F

Use The initials of each day to track Your New & Old Habits

Water Intake	64oz. 's
Monday	
Tuesday	
Wednesday	
Thursday	
Friday	
Saturday	
Sunday	

Weekly Menu

Monday:

Tuesday:

Wednesday:

Thursday:

Friday:

Weekend:

Saturday	Sunday

Exercise/ 🏋 Cardio 🏃	🕐
Monday	
Tuesday	
Wednesday	
Thursday	
Friday	
Saturday	
Sunday	

Specify whether Cardio or Strength Training. E/C

Put a check mark if you ate on time!	Brkfast	Lunch	Dinner
Monday	🎭		
Tuesday	✓		
Wednesday			
Thursday			
Friday			
Saturday			
Sunday			

🎭 1 hr After each meal write an emoji for how you feel as far as energy, happy for good sad for bad!

Habit Tracker

Positive Pick New	Negative Pick Old
T	
W	F

Use The initials of each day to track Your New & Old Habits

Water Intake	64oz. 's
Monday	
Tuesday	
Wednesday	
Thursday	
Friday	
Saturday	
Sunday	

Exercise/ Cardio	
Monday	
Tuesday	
Wednesday	
Thursday	
Friday	
Saturday	
Sunday	

Specify whether Cardio or Strength Training. E/C

Weekly Menu

Monday:

Tuesday:

Wednesday:

Thursday:

Friday:

Weekend:

Saturday	Sunday

Put a check mark if you ate on time!	Brkfast	Lunch	Dinner
Monday	🎭		
Tuesday	✓		
Wednesday			
Thursday			
Friday			
Saturday			
Sunday			

🎭 1 hr After each meal write an emoji for how you feel as far as energy, happy for good sad for bad!

Habit Tracker

Positive Pick New		Negative Pick Old	
T			
W		F	

Use The initials of each day to track Your New & Old Habits

Water Intake	64oz. 's
Monday	
Tuesday	
Wednesday	
Thursday	
Friday	
Saturday	
Sunday	

Exercise/ Cardio 🏋🚶 🕐	
Monday	
Tuesday	
Wednesday	
Thursday	
Friday	
Saturday	
Sunday	

Specify whether Cardio or Strength Training. E/C

Weekly Menu

Monday:

Tuesday:

Wednesday:

Thursday:

Friday:

Weekend:

Saturday	Sunday

Put a check mark if you ate on time!	Brkfast	Lunch	Dinner
Monday	🎭		
Tuesday	✓		
Wednesday			
Thursday			
Friday			
Saturday			
Sunday			

🎭 1 hr After each meal write an emoji for how you feel as far as energy, happy for good sad for bad!

Habit Tracker

Positive Pick New	Negative Pick Old
T	
W	F

Use The initials of each day to track Your New & Old Habits

Water Intake	64oz. 's
Monday	
Tuesday	
Wednesday	
Thursday	
Friday	
Saturday	
Sunday	

Exercise/Cardio	
Monday	
Tuesday	
Wednesday	
Thursday	
Friday	
Saturday	
Sunday	

Specify whether Cardio or Strength Training. E/C

Weekly Menu

Monday:

Tuesday:

Wednesday:

Thursday:

Friday:

Weekend:

Saturday	Sunday

Put a check mark if you ate on time!	Brkfast	Lunch	Dinner
Monday	🎭		
Tuesday	✓		
Wednesday			
Thursday			
Friday			
Saturday			
Sunday			

🎭 1 hr After each meal write an emoji for how you feel as far as energy, happy for good sad for bad!

Habit Tracker

Positive Pick New	Negative Pick Old
T	
W	F

Use The initials of each day to track Your New & Old Habits

Water Intake	64oz. 🥛's
Monday	
Tuesday	
Wednesday	
Thursday	
Friday	
Saturday	
Sunday	

Exercise/ Cardio 🏋️🚶	🕐
Monday	
Tuesday	
Wednesday	
Thursday	
Friday	
Saturday	
Sunday	

Specify whether Cardio or Strength Training. E/C

Weekly Menu

Monday:

Tuesday:

Wednesday:

Thursday:

Friday:

Weekend:

Saturday	Sunday

August 2020

Sun	Mon	Tue	Wed	Thu	Fri	Sat
	27	28	29	30	31	1
2	3	4	5	6	7	8
9	10	11	12	13	14	15
16	17	18	19	20	21	22
23	24	25	26	27	28	29
30	31	1	2	3	4	5

Monthly Overview/Notes
_____
_____
_____
_____

Put a check mark if you ate on time!	Brkfast	Lunch	Dinner
Monday	🎭		
Tuesday	✓		
Wednesday			
Thursday			
Friday			
Saturday			
Sunday			

🎭 1 hr After each meal write an emoji for how you feel as far as energy, happy for good sad for bad!

Habit Tracker

Positive Pick New	Negative Pick Old
T	
W	F

Use The initials of each day to track Your New & Old Habits

Water Intake	64oz. 's
Monday	
Tuesday	
Wednesday	
Thursday	
Friday	
Saturday	
Sunday	

Exercise/ Cardio 🏋️🏃 🕒	
Monday	
Tuesday	
Wednesday	
Thursday	
Friday	
Saturday	
Sunday	

Specify whether Cardio or Strength Training. E/C

Weekly Menu

Monday:

Tuesday:

Wednesday:

Thursday:

Friday:

Weekend:

Saturday	Sunday

Put a check mark if you ate on time!	Brkfast	Lunch	Dinner
Monday	🎭		
Tuesday	✓		
Wednesday			
Thursday			
Friday			
Saturday			
Sunday			

🎭🎭 1 hr After each meal write an emoji for how you feel as far as energy, happy for good sad for bad!

Habit Tracker

Positive Pick New	Negative Pick Old
T	
W	F

Use The initials of each day to track Your New & Old Habits

Water Intake	64oz. 's
Monday	
Tuesday	
Wednesday	
Thursday	
Friday	
Saturday	
Sunday	

Exercise/ Cardio	
Monday	
Tuesday	
Wednesday	
Thursday	
Friday	
Saturday	
Sunday	

Specify whether Cardio or Strength Training. E/C

Weekly Menu

Monday:

Tuesday:

Wednesday:

Thursday:

Friday:

Weekend:

Saturday	Sunday

What are some New foods you can try make a list?	Brkfast	Lunch	Dinner
Monday			
Tuesday			
Wednesday			
Thursday			
Friday			
Saturday			
Sunday			

1 hr After each meal mark how you feel as far as energy, with the New Foods from Your list!

New Habits

What are some New things that You would like to try?
1. _____
2. _____
3. _____

Okay Pick one & Track

M	T	W	Th	F	S	S

Put a check mark each day to track Your New Habit for the next 6 Weeks

Water Intake	64oz. 's
Week 35	
Week 36	
Week 37	
Week 38	
Week 39	

Did you drink at least 64 oz. of water every day each week?

Exercise/ Cardio	E	C
Week 35		
Week 36		
Week 37		
Week 38		
Week 39		

Fill in how many hours You Trained for each week

Progress Assessment

1-10 How do I feel about my progress?

How many pounds have I lost?

How many inches have I lost?

How do I look in the mirror?

What size is my clothing now?

Have I bought new clothes yet?

How has my energy been lately?

How have my workouts been?

How have you been in regards to health?

What do you like most, the way you feel or look? Why?

What do I enjoy most, exercise or eating healthy?

Who is one person that you can support to get healthy?

Who do you need to stay away from & Why?

Put a check mark if you ate on time!	Brkfast	Lunch	Dinner
Monday	🎭		
Tuesday	✓		
Wednesday			
Thursday			
Friday			
Saturday			
Sunday			

🎭 1 hr After each meal write an emoji for how you feel as far as energy, happy for good sad for bad!

Habit Tracker

Positive Pick New	Negative Pick Old
T	
W	F

Use The initials of each day to track Your New & Old Habits

Water Intake	64oz. 's
Monday	
Tuesday	
Wednesday	
Thursday	
Friday	
Saturday	
Sunday	

Weekly Menu

Monday:

Tuesday:

Wednesday:

Thursday:

Friday:

Weekend:

Saturday	Sunday

Exercise/ Cardio 🏋🏃🕒	
Monday	
Tuesday	
Wednesday	
Thursday	
Friday	
Saturday	
Sunday	

Specify whether Cardio or Strength Training. E/C

Put a check mark if you ate on time!	Brkfast	Lunch	Dinner
Monday	🎭		
Tuesday	✓		
Wednesday			
Thursday			
Friday			
Saturday			
Sunday			

🎭 1 hr After each meal write an emoji for how you feel as far as energy, happy for good sad for bad!

Habit Tracker

Positive Pick New			Negative Pick Old		
	T				
W					F

Use The initials of each day to track Your New & Old Habits

Water Intake	64oz. 🥛 's
Monday	
Tuesday	
Wednesday	
Thursday	
Friday	
Saturday	
Sunday	

Exercise/ Cardio 🏋🏃 🕐	
Monday	
Tuesday	
Wednesday	
Thursday	
Friday	
Saturday	
Sunday	

Specify whether Cardio or Strength Training. E/C

Weekly Menu

Monday:

Tuesday:

Wednesday:

Thursday:

Friday:

Weekend:

Saturday	Sunday

Put a check mark if you ate on time!	Brkfast	Lunch	Dinner
Monday	🎭		
Tuesday	✓		
Wednesday			
Thursday			
Friday			
Saturday			
Sunday			

1 hr After each meal write an emoji for how you feel as far as energy, happy for good sad for bad!

Habit Tracker

Positive Pick New	Negative Pick Old
T	
W	F

Use The initials of each day to track Your New & Old Habits

Water Intake	64oz. 🥛's
Monday	
Tuesday	
Wednesday	
Thursday	
Friday	
Saturday	
Sunday	

Exercise/Cardio		
Monday		
Tuesday		
Wednesday		
Thursday		
Friday		
Saturday		
Sunday		

Specify whether Cardio or Strength Training. E/C

Weekly Menu

Monday:

Tuesday:

Wednesday:

Thursday:

Friday:

Weekend:

Saturday	Sunday

September 2020

Sun	Mon	Tue	Wed	Thu	Fri	Sat
	31	1	2	3	4	5
6	7 Labor	8	9	10	11	12
13	14	15	16	17	18 Air Force	19 Rosh Has.
20	21	22	23	24	25	26
27	28 Yom Kip.	29	30	1	2	3

Monthly Overview/Notes

_____
_____
_____
_____

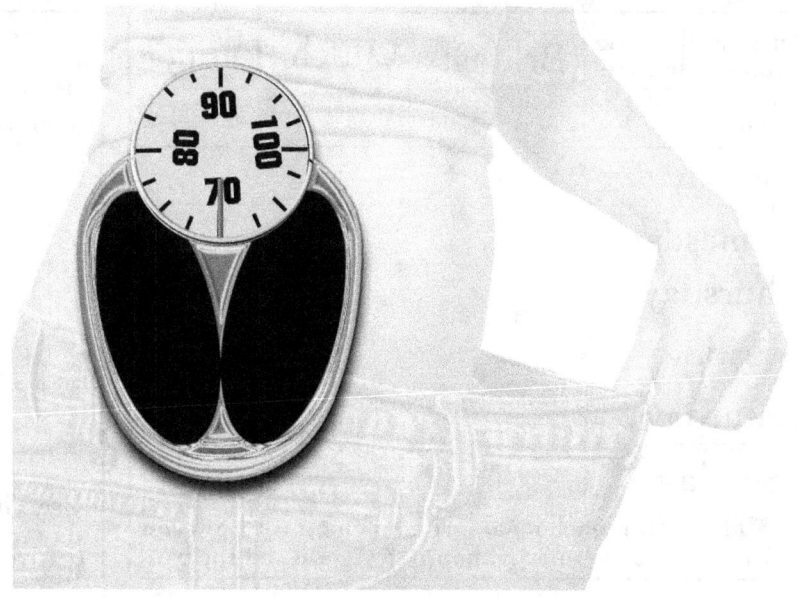

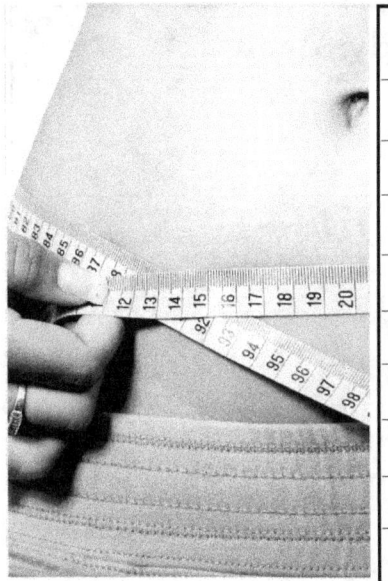

Measurements

Weight		Body Mass Index (BMI)	
Body Fat %		Water Weight	
Bust		Muscle Weight	
Chest		**Notes**	
Waist			
Hips			
Thighs			
Calves			
Upper Arm			
Fore Arm			

Do you notice anything new energy, feelings, etc?

Ok it's been a while how faithful have you been?

Are you happy with your progress so far?

Have you been loving or neglecting yourself??? Why?

Put a check mark if you ate on time!	Brkfast	Lunch	Dinner
Monday	🎭		
Tuesday	✓		
Wednesday			
Thursday			
Friday			
Saturday			
Sunday			

🎭 1 hr After each meal write an emoji for how you feel as far as energy, happy for good sad for bad!

Habit Tracker

Positive Pick New	Negative Pick Old
T	
W	F

Use The initials of each day to track Your New & Old Habits

Water Intake	64oz. 🥛's
Monday	
Tuesday	
Wednesday	
Thursday	
Friday	
Saturday	
Sunday	

Exercise/Cardio 🏋️🏃 🕒	
Monday	
Tuesday	
Wednesday	
Thursday	
Friday	
Saturday	
Sunday	

Specify whether Cardio or Strength Training. E/C

Weekly Menu

Monday:

Tuesday:

Wednesday:

Thursday:

Friday:

Weekend:

Saturday	Sunday

Put a check mark if you ate on time!	Brkfast	Lunch	Dinner
Monday	🎭		
Tuesday	✓		
Wednesday			
Thursday			
Friday			
Saturday			
Sunday			

🎭 1 hr After each meal write an emoji for how you feel as far as energy, happy for good sad for bad!

Habit Tracker

Positive Pick New	Negative Pick Old
T	
W	F

Use The initials of each day to track Your New & Old Habits

Water Intake	64oz. 's
Monday	
Tuesday	
Wednesday	
Thursday	
Friday	
Saturday	
Sunday	

Exercise/ Cardio 🏋️ 🚶 🕒	
Monday	
Tuesday	
Wednesday	
Thursday	
Friday	
Saturday	
Sunday	

Specify whether Cardio or Strength Training. E/C

Weekly Menu

Monday:

Tuesday:

Wednesday:

Thursday:

Friday:

Weekend:

Saturday	Sunday

Put a check mark if you ate on time!	Brkfast	Lunch	Dinner
Monday	🎭		
Tuesday	✓		
Wednesday			
Thursday			
Friday			
Saturday			
Sunday			

🎭 1 hr After each meal write an emoji for how you feel as far as energy, happy for good sad for bad!

Habit Tracker

Positive Pick New		Negative Pick Old	
T			
W			F

Use The initials of each day to track Your New & Old Habits

Water Intake	64oz. 🥛's
Monday	
Tuesday	
Wednesday	
Thursday	
Friday	
Saturday	
Sunday	

Weekly Menu

Monday:

Tuesday:

Wednesday:

Thursday:

Friday:

Weekend:

Saturday	Sunday

Exercise/ Cardio 🏃	🕒
Monday	
Tuesday	
Wednesday	
Thursday	
Friday	
Saturday	
Sunday	

Specify whether Cardio or Strength Training. E/C

Put a check mark if you ate on time!	Brkfast	Lunch	Dinner
Monday	🎭		
Tuesday	✓		
Wednesday			
Thursday			
Friday			
Saturday			
Sunday			

🎭 1 hr After each meal write an emoji for how you feel as far as energy, happy for good sad for bad!

Habit Tracker

Positive Pick New	Negative Pick Old
T	
W	F

Use The initials of each day to track Your New & Old Habits

Water Intake	64oz. 's
Monday	
Tuesday	
Wednesday	
Thursday	
Friday	
Saturday	
Sunday	

Weekly Menu

Monday:

Tuesday:

Wednesday:

Thursday:

Friday:

Weekend:

Saturday	Sunday

Exercise/ Cardio 🏃 🏋️	🕐
Monday	
Tuesday	
Wednesday	
Thursday	
Friday	
Saturday	
Sunday	

Specify whether Cardio or Strength Training. E/C

Put a check mark if you ate on time!	Brkfast	Lunch	Dinner
Monday	🎭		
Tuesday	✓		
Wednesday			
Thursday			
Friday			
Saturday			
Sunday			

🎭 1 hr After each meal write an emoji for how you feel as far as energy, happy for good sad for bad!

Habit Tracker

Positive Pick New		Negative Pick Old	
	T		
W			F

Use The initials of each day to track Your New & Old Habits

Water Intake	64oz. 🥤 's
Monday	
Tuesday	
Wednesday	
Thursday	
Friday	
Saturday	
Sunday	

Weekly Menu

Monday:

Tuesday:

Wednesday:

Thursday:

Friday:

Weekend:

Saturday	Sunday

Exercise/ Cardio 🏋️🏃 🕐	
Monday	
Tuesday	
Wednesday	
Thursday	
Friday	
Saturday	
Sunday	

Specify whether Cardio or Strength Training. E/C

October 2020

Sun	Mon	Tue	Wed	Thu	Fri	Sat
	28	29	30	1	2	3 **1st. D Suk**
4	5	6	7	8	9 **Last Suk.**	10 **Shm.Atz**
11 **Sim.Tor**	12 **Columbus**	13 **Navy**	14	15	16	17
18	19	20	21	22	23	24
25	26	27	28	29	30	31 **Halloween**

Monthly Overview/Notes

_____
_____
_____
_____

Put a check mark if you ate on time!	Brkfast	Lunch	Dinner
Monday	🎭		
Tuesday	✓		
Wednesday			
Thursday			
Friday			
Saturday			
Sunday			

🎭 1 hr After each meal write an emoji for how you feel as far as energy, happy for good sad for bad!

Habit Tracker

Positive Pick New	Negative Pick Old
T	
W	F

Use The initials of each day to track Your New & Old Habits

Water Intake	64oz. 🥤's
Monday	
Tuesday	
Wednesday	
Thursday	
Friday	
Saturday	
Sunday	

Exercise/ Cardio 🏋️🏃	🕐
Monday	
Tuesday	
Wednesday	
Thursday	
Friday	
Saturday	
Sunday	

Specify whether Cardio or Strength Training. E/C

Weekly Menu

Monday:

Tuesday:

Wednesday:

Thursday:

Friday:

Weekend:

Saturday	Sunday

Put a check mark if you ate on time!	Brkfast	Lunch	Dinner
Monday	🎭		
Tuesday	✓		
Wednesday			
Thursday			
Friday			
Saturday			
Sunday			

🎭 1 hr After each meal write an emoji for how you feel as far as energy, happy for good sad for bad!

Habit Tracker

Positive Pick New	Negative Pick Old
T	
W	F

Use The initials of each day to track Your New & Old Habits

Water Intake	64oz. 🥛's
Monday	
Tuesday	
Wednesday	
Thursday	
Friday	
Saturday	
Sunday	

Exercise/ 🏋️ Cardio 🏃 🕐	
Monday	
Tuesday	
Wednesday	
Thursday	
Friday	
Saturday	
Sunday	

Specify whether Cardio or Strength Training. E/C

Weekly Menu

Monday:

Tuesday:

Wednesday:

Thursday:

Friday:

Weekend:

Saturday	Sunday

Put a check mark if you ate on time!	Brkfast	Lunch	Dinner
Monday	🎭		
Tuesday	✓		
Wednesday			
Thursday			
Friday			
Saturday			
Sunday			

🎭 1 hr After each meal write an emoji for how you feel as far as energy, happy for good sad for bad!

Habit Tracker	
Positive Pick New	Negative Pick Old
T	
W	F

Use The initials of each day to track Your New & Old Habits

Water Intake	64oz. 's
Monday	
Tuesday	
Wednesday	
Thursday	
Friday	
Saturday	
Sunday	

Exercise/ Cardio 🏋🏃 🕐	
Monday	
Tuesday	
Wednesday	
Thursday	
Friday	
Saturday	
Sunday	

Specify whether Cardio or Strength Training. E/C

Weekly Menu

Monday:

Tuesday:

Wednesday:

Thursday:

Friday:

Weekend:

Saturday	Sunday

Put a check mark if you ate on time!	Brkfast	Lunch	Dinner
Monday	🎭		
Tuesday	✓		
Wednesday			
Thursday			
Friday			
Saturday			
Sunday			

🎭 1 hr After each meal write an emoji for how you feel as far as energy, happy for good sad for bad!

Habit Tracker

Positive Pick New	Negative Pick Old
T	
W	F

Use The initials of each day to track Your New & Old Habits

Water Intake	64oz. 's
Monday	
Tuesday	
Wednesday	
Thursday	
Friday	
Saturday	
Sunday	

Weekly Menu

Monday:

Tuesday:

Wednesday:

Thursday:

Friday:

Weekend:

Saturday	Sunday

Exercise/ Cardio	
Monday	
Tuesday	
Wednesday	
Thursday	
Friday	
Saturday	
Sunday	

Specify whether Cardio or Strength Training. E/C

Put a check mark if you ate on time!	Brkfast	Lunch	Dinner
Monday	🎭		
Tuesday	✓		
Wednesday			
Thursday			
Friday			
Saturday			
Sunday			

🎭 1 hr After each meal write an emoji for how you feel as far as energy, happy for good sad for bad!

Habit Tracker

Positive Pick New	Negative Pick Old
T	
W	F

Use The initials of each day to track Your New & Old Habits

Water Intake	64oz. 's
Monday	
Tuesday	
Wednesday	
Thursday	
Friday	
Saturday	
Sunday	

Exercise/ Cardio 🏋🏃 🕒	
Monday	
Tuesday	
Wednesday	
Thursday	
Friday	
Saturday	
Sunday	

Specify whether Cardio or Strength Training. E/C

Weekly Menu

Monday:

Tuesday:

Wednesday:

Thursday:

Friday:

Weekend:

Saturday	Sunday

November 2020

Sun	Mon	Tue	Wed	Thu	Fri	Sat
1 DLS	2	3 Election	4	5	6	7
8	9	10	11 Veterans	12	13	14
15	16	17	18	19	20	21
22	23	24	25	26 Thanks Giving	27 Black Friday	28
29	30 Cyber Monday	1	2	3	4	

Monthly Overview/Notes

_____
_____
_____
_____

Put a check mark if you ate on time!	Brkfast	Lunch	Dinner
Monday	🎭		
Tuesday	✓		
Wednesday			
Thursday			
Friday			
Saturday			
Sunday			

🎭 1 hr After each meal write an emoji for how you feel as far as energy, happy for good sad for bad!

Habit Tracker

Positive Pick New	Negative Pick Old
T	
W	F

Use The initials of each day to track Your New & Old Habits

Water Intake	64oz. 🥛's
Monday	
Tuesday	
Wednesday	
Thursday	
Friday	
Saturday	
Sunday	

Exercise/ Cardio 🏋️🏃 🕒	
Monday	
Tuesday	
Wednesday	
Thursday	
Friday	
Saturday	
Sunday	

Specify whether Cardio or Strength Training. E/C

Weekly Menu

Monday:

Tuesday:

Wednesday:

Thursday:

Friday:

Weekend:

Saturday	Sunday

Put a check mark if you ate on time!	Brkfast	Lunch	Dinner
Monday	🎭		
Tuesday	✓		
Wednesday			
Thursday			
Friday			
Saturday			
Sunday			

🎭🎭 1 hr After each meal write an emoji for how you feel as far as energy, happy for good sad for bad!

Habit Tracker

Positive Pick New	Negative Pick Old
T	
W	F

Use The initials of each day to track Your New & Old Habits

Water Intake	64oz. 🥛 's
Monday	
Tuesday	
Wednesday	
Thursday	
Friday	
Saturday	
Sunday	

Exercise/ 🏋️ Cardio 🏃 🕐	
Monday	
Tuesday	
Wednesday	
Thursday	
Friday	
Saturday	
Sunday	

Specify whether Cardio or Strength Training. E/C

Weekly Menu

Monday:

Tuesday:

Wednesday:

Thursday:

Friday:

Weekend:

Saturday	Sunday

Put a check mark if you ate on time!	Brkfast	Lunch	Dinner
Monday	🎭		
Tuesday	✓		
Wednesday			
Thursday			
Friday			
Saturday			
Sunday			

🎭 1 hr After each meal write an emoji for how you feel as far as energy, happy for good sad for bad!

Habit Tracker

Positive Pick New	Negative Pick Old
T	
W	F

Use The initials of each day to track Your New & Old Habits

Water Intake	64oz. 🥤 's
Monday	
Tuesday	
Wednesday	
Thursday	
Friday	
Saturday	
Sunday	

Exercise/ 🏋 Cardio 🚶	🕒
Monday	
Tuesday	
Wednesday	
Thursday	
Friday	
Saturday	
Sunday	

Specify whether Cardio or Strength Training. E/C

Weekly Menu

Monday:

Tuesday:

Wednesday:

Thursday:

Friday:

Weekend:

Saturday	Sunday

Put a check mark if you ate on time!	Brkfast	Lunch	Dinner
Monday	🎭		
Tuesday	✓		
Wednesday			
Thursday			
Friday			
Saturday			
Sunday			

🎭 1 hr After each meal write an emoji for how you feel as far as energy, happy for good sad for bad!

Habit Tracker

Positive Pick New	Negative Pick Old
T	
W	F

Use The initials of each day to track Your New & Old Habits

Water Intake	64oz. 's
Monday	
Tuesday	
Wednesday	
Thursday	
Friday	
Saturday	
Sunday	

Weekly Menu

Monday:

Tuesday:

Wednesday:

Thursday:

Friday:

Weekend:

Saturday	Sunday

Exercise/ Cardio 🏋️🏃 🕐	
Monday	
Tuesday	
Wednesday	
Thursday	
Friday	
Saturday	
Sunday	

Specify whether Cardio or Strength Training. E/C

What are some New foods you can try make a list?	Brkfast	Lunch	Dinner
Monday			
Tuesday			
Wednesday			
Thursday			
Friday			
Saturday			
Sunday			

1 hr After each meal mark how you feel as far as energy, with the New Foods from Your list!

New Habits

What are some New things that You would like to try?
1.
2.
3.

Okay Pick one & Track

M	T	W	Th	F	S	S

Put a check mark each day to track Your New Habit for the next 6 Weeks

Water Intake	64oz. 's
Week 45	
Week 46	
Week 47	
Week 48	
Week 49	

Have you been keeping up with your water intake?

Exercise/ Cardio	E	C
Week 45		
Week 46		
Week 47		
Week 48		
Week 49		

Fill in how many hours You Trained for each week

Progress Assessment

1-10 How do I feel about my progress?

How many pounds have I lost?

How many inches have I lost around my waist?

How do you look in the mirror on a scale of 1-10?

What size is your clothing now?

How has your energy been lately?

Have you been sticking to your workouts? Why?

Who have been your best Supporters?

What has been the hardest part of this journey?

What do you like most about where you are today?

December 2020

Sun	Mon	Tue	Wed	Thu	Fri	Sat
	30	1 **RosaParks**	2	3	4	5
6	7	8	9	10	11 **Hanukkah**	12
13	14	15	16	17	18 **Han.Ends**	19
20	21	22	23	24	25 **Christmas**	26 **Kwanzaa**
27	28	29	30	31	1 **New Years**	2

Monthly Overview/Notes

_____
_____
_____
_____

Put a check mark if you ate on time!	Brkfast	Lunch	Dinner
Monday	🎭		
Tuesday	✓		
Wednesday			
Thursday			
Friday			
Saturday			
Sunday			

🎭 1 hr After each meal write an emoji for how you feel as far as energy, happy for good sad for bad!

Habit Tracker

Positive Pick New	Negative Pick Old
T	
W	F

Use The initials of each day to track Your New & Old Habits

Water Intake	64oz. 's
Monday	
Tuesday	
Wednesday	
Thursday	
Friday	
Saturday	
Sunday	

Exercise/ Cardio 🏋️🏃 🕐	
Monday	
Tuesday	
Wednesday	
Thursday	
Friday	
Saturday	
Sunday	

Specify whether Cardio or Strength Training. E/C

Weekly Menu

Monday:

Tuesday:

Wednesday:

Thursday:

Friday:

Weekend:

Saturday	Sunday

Put a check mark if you ate on time!	Brkfast	Lunch	Dinner
Monday	🎭		
Tuesday	✓		
Wednesday			
Thursday			
Friday			
Saturday			
Sunday			

🎭 1 hr After each meal write an emoji for how you feel as far as energy, happy for good sad for bad!

Habit Tracker

Positive Pick New	Negative Pick Old
T	
W	F

Use The initials of each day to track Your New & Old Habits

Water Intake	64oz. 's
Monday	
Tuesday	
Wednesday	
Thursday	
Friday	
Saturday	
Sunday	

Exercise/ Cardio 🏃 🏋 🕐	
Monday	
Tuesday	
Wednesday	
Thursday	
Friday	
Saturday	
Sunday	

Specify whether Cardio or Strength Training. E/C

Weekly Menu

Monday:

Tuesday:

Wednesday:

Thursday:

Friday:

Weekend:

Saturday	Sunday

Put a check mark if you ate on time!	Brkfast	Lunch	Dinner
Monday	🎭		
Tuesday	✓		
Wednesday			
Thursday			
Friday			
Saturday			
Sunday			

🎭 1 hr After each meal write an emoji for how you feel as far as energy, happy for good sad for bad!

Habit Tracker

Positive Pick New	Negative Pick Old
T	
W	F

Use The initials of each day to track Your New & Old Habits

Water Intake	64oz. 's
Monday	
Tuesday	
Wednesday	
Thursday	
Friday	
Saturday	
Sunday	

Exercise/ Cardio 🏋🚶 🕒	
Monday	
Tuesday	
Wednesday	
Thursday	
Friday	
Saturday	
Sunday	

Specify whether Cardio or Strength Training. E/C

Weekly Menu

Monday:

Tuesday:

Wednesday:

Thursday:

Friday:

Weekend:

Saturday	Sunday

Put a check mark if you ate on time!	Brkfast	Lunch	Dinner
Monday	🎭		
Tuesday	✓		
Wednesday			
Thursday			
Friday			
Saturday			
Sunday			

🎭🎭 1 hr After each meal write an emoji for how you feel as far as energy, happy for good sad for bad!

Habit Tracker

Positive Pick New	Negative Pick Old
T	
W	F

Use The initials of each day to track Your New & Old Habits

Water Intake	64oz. 's
Monday	
Tuesday	
Wednesday	
Thursday	
Friday	
Saturday	
Sunday	

Exercise/ Cardio	🏋️ 🕐
Monday	
Tuesday	
Wednesday	
Thursday	
Friday	
Saturday	
Sunday	

Specify whether Cardio or Strength Training. E/C

Weekly Menu

Monday:

Tuesday:

Wednesday:

Thursday:

Friday:

Weekend:

Saturday	Sunday

Put a check mark if you ate on time!	Brkfast	Lunch	Dinner
Monday	🎭		
Tuesday	✓		
Wednesday			
Thursday			
Friday			
Saturday			
Sunday			

🎭 1 hr After each meal write an emoji for how you feel as far as energy, happy for good sad for bad!

Habit Tracker

Positive Pick New	Negative Pick Old
T	
W	F

Use The initials of each day to track Your New & Old Habits

Water Intake	64oz. 's
Monday	
Tuesday	
Wednesday	
Thursday	
Friday	
Saturday	
Sunday	

Exercise/ Cardio 🏋🚶	🕐
Monday	
Tuesday	
Wednesday	
Thursday	
Friday	
Saturday	
Sunday	

Specify whether Cardio or Strength Training. E/C

Weekly Menu

Monday:

Tuesday:

Wednesday:

Thursday:

Friday:

Weekend:

Saturday	Sunday

MY
Reasons Why I Love
My
Self
JOURNAL

Because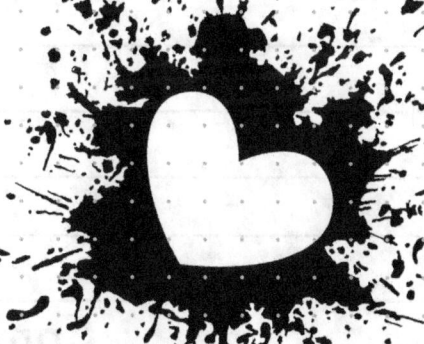

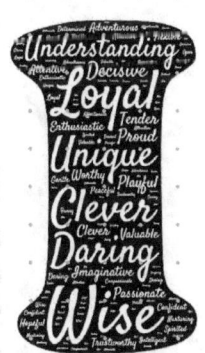 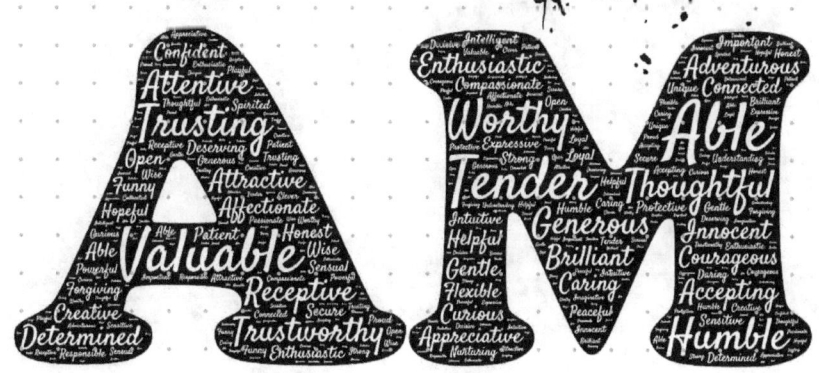

Comments/Notes

Comments/Notes

Comments/Notes

Comments/Notes

Comments/Notes

Comments/Notes

Comments/Notes

Comments/Notes

Comments/Notes

Comments/Notes

Comments/Notes

Comments/Notes

Comments/Notes

Comments/Notes

Comments/Notes

Comments/Notes

Comments/Notes

Comments/Notes

Comments/Notes

Comments/Notes

Comments/Notes

Comments/Notes

Comments/Notes

Comments/Notes

Comments/Notes

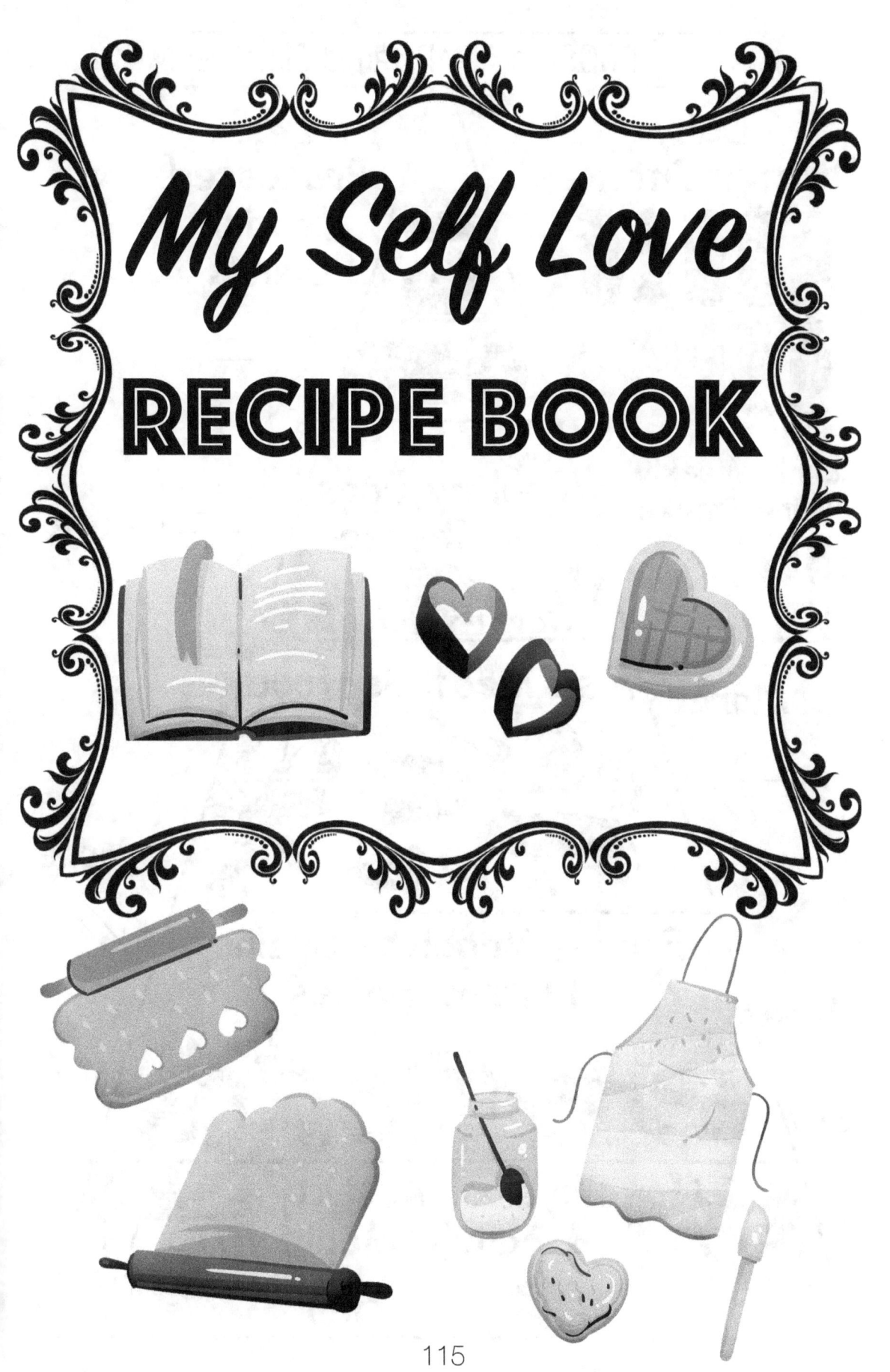

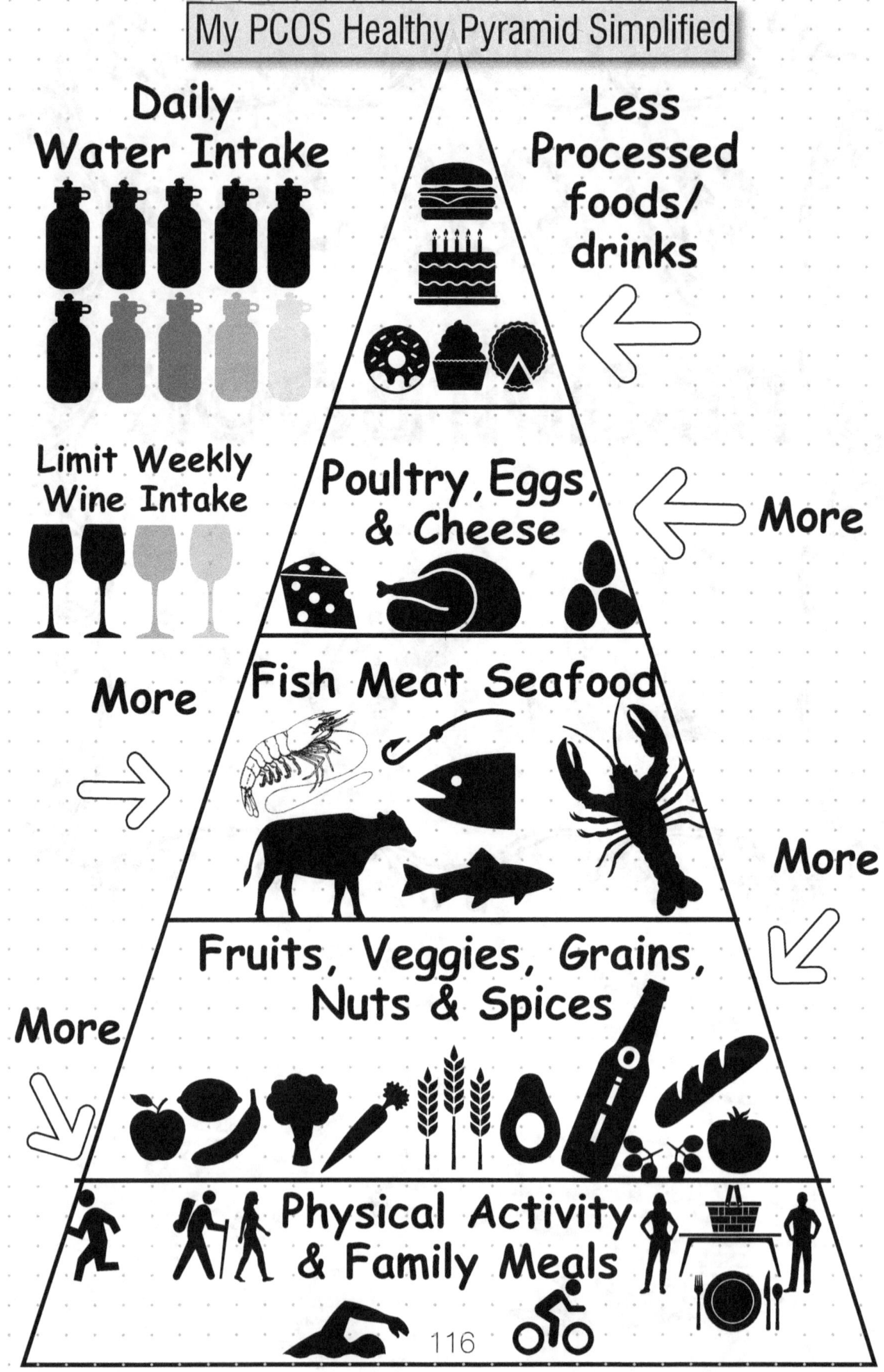

Fruit & Vegetable Starter List
6-8 per day

Apples	Broccoli	Avocado	Artichokes
Apricots	Carrots	Berries	Beets
Bananas	Cucumbers	Clementines	Cabbage
Cherries	Eggplant	Bananas	Greens
Dates	Melons	Cherries	Onions
Figs	Peaches	Pears	Pears
Grapes	Turnips	Peppers	Peas
Oranges	Yams	Tomatoes	Zucchini

Seafood & Fish Starter List

Mackerel	Herring	Clams
Bass	Mahi-mahi	Crabs
Cod	Salmon	Lobster
King Fish	Sardines	Mussels
Perch	Shark	Oysters
Pollock	Tuna	Scallops
Swordfish	Trout	Shrimp
	Snapper	

Herbs & Spices Starter List

Basil
Coriander
Cumin
Garlic
Mint
Rosemary
Sage
Tarragon

Allspice
Cinnamon
Nutmeg
Oregano
Parsley
Spanish Paprika

Cardamom
Cilantro
Thyme
Turmeric
Saffron
Sumac
Za'atar

Healthy Fats & Oils Starter List

3-5 x per day	3-5 x per day	1-2 x per day
Olives/Oil Nut/Butters/Oils Fish/Oils Seed/Oils	Avocado/Oils/Butters Coconut/MCT Oil	Yogurts Ghee Cottage Cheese

If you drink milk make it Almond (yes it's processed but you're not a calf so NO cow's milk) or something similar like rice or something.

Healthy Grains Starter List

Bulgar	*Brown Rice*	*Rye*
Buckwheat	*Barley*	*Popcorn*
Oats	*Couscous*	*Sorghum*
Farro	*Millet*	*Maize*
Polenta	*Quinoa*	*Whole Grain*
Wheat Berries	*Spelt*	*Wild Rice*

Recipe: _____

Serving: _____   Prep Time: _____

Cook Time: _____ Temperature: _____

Ingredients: Methods:
_____   _____
_____   _____
_____   _____
_____   _____
_____   _____
_____   _____
_____   _____
_____   _____
_____   _____
_____   _____
_____   _____
_____   _____
_____   _____
_____   _____
_____   _____

Notes

_____
_____
_____

Recipe: _____

Serving: _____   Prep Time: _____

Cook Time: _____   Temperature: _____

Ingredients: Methods:

_____   _____
_____   _____
_____   _____
_____   _____
_____   _____
_____   _____
_____   _____
_____   _____
_____   _____
_____   _____
_____   _____
_____   _____
_____   _____
_____   _____
_____   _____
_____   _____
_____   _____

Notes

_____
_____
_____

Recipe: _____

Serving: _____   Prep Time: _____

Cook Time: _____   Temperature: _____

Ingredients: Methods:
_____   _____
_____   _____
_____   _____
_____   _____
_____   _____
_____   _____
_____   _____
_____   _____
_____   _____
_____   _____
_____   _____
_____   _____
_____   _____
_____   _____
_____   _____
_____   _____
_____   _____
_____   _____

Notes

_____
_____
_____

Recipe: _____

Serving: _____   Prep Time: _____

Cook Time: _____   Temperature: _____

Ingredients:

_____
_____
_____
_____
_____
_____
_____
_____
_____
_____
_____
_____
_____
_____
_____
_____
_____
_____

Methods:

_____
_____
_____
_____
_____
_____
_____
_____
_____
_____
_____
_____
_____
_____
_____
_____
_____
_____

Notes

_____
_____
_____

Recipe: _____

Serving: _____ Prep Time: _____

Cook Time: _____ Temperature: _____

Ingredients:

_____
_____
_____
_____
_____
_____
_____
_____
_____
_____
_____
_____
_____
_____
_____
_____
_____
_____
_____

Methods:

_____
_____
_____
_____
_____
_____
_____
_____
_____
_____
_____
_____
_____
_____
_____
_____
_____
_____
_____

Notes

_____
_____
_____

Recipe: _____

Serving: _____   Prep Time: _____

Cook Time: _____   Temperature: _____

Ingredients:

_____
_____
_____
_____
_____
_____
_____
_____
_____
_____
_____
_____
_____
_____
_____
_____
_____
_____
_____

Methods:

_____
_____
_____
_____
_____
_____
_____
_____
_____
_____
_____
_____
_____
_____
_____
_____
_____
_____
_____

Notes

_____
_____
_____

Recipe: _____

Serving: _____   Prep Time: _____

Cook Time: _____   Temperature: _____

Ingredients:

_____
_____
_____
_____
_____
_____
_____
_____
_____
_____
_____
_____
_____
_____
_____
_____
_____
_____
_____

Methods:

_____
_____
_____
_____
_____
_____
_____
_____
_____
_____
_____
_____
_____
_____
_____
_____
_____
_____
_____

Notes

_____
_____
_____

Recipe: _____

Serving: _____   Prep Time: _____

Cook Time: _____   Temperature: _____

Ingredients: Methods:
_____   _____
_____   _____
_____   _____
_____   _____
_____   _____
_____   _____
_____   _____
_____   _____
_____   _____
_____   _____
_____   _____
_____   _____
_____   _____
_____   _____
_____   _____
_____   _____

Notes
_____
_____

Recipe: _____

Serving: _____ Prep Time: _____

Cook Time: _____ Temperature: _____

Ingredients:

_____
_____
_____
_____
_____
_____
_____
_____
_____
_____
_____
_____
_____
_____
_____
_____
_____

Methods:

_____
_____
_____
_____
_____
_____
_____
_____
_____
_____
_____
_____
_____
_____
_____
_____
_____

Notes

_____
_____
_____

Recipe: _____

Serving: _____   Prep Time: _____

Cook Time: _____   Temperature: _____

Ingredients:

_____
_____
_____
_____
_____
_____
_____
_____
_____
_____
_____
_____
_____
_____
_____
_____
_____
_____
_____

Methods:

_____
_____
_____
_____
_____
_____
_____
_____
_____
_____
_____
_____
_____
_____
_____
_____
_____
_____
_____

Notes

_____
_____
_____

Recipe: _____

Serving: _____   Prep Time: _____

Cook Time: _____   Temperature: _____

Ingredients:

_____
_____
_____
_____
_____
_____
_____
_____
_____
_____
_____
_____
_____
_____
_____
_____
_____

Methods:

_____
_____
_____
_____
_____
_____
_____
_____
_____
_____
_____
_____
_____
_____
_____
_____
_____

Notes

_____
_____
_____

Recipe: _____

Serving: _____   Prep Time: _____

Cook Time: _____   Temperature: _____

Ingredients: Methods:

_____   _____
_____   _____
_____   _____
_____   _____
_____   _____
_____   _____
_____   _____
_____   _____
_____   _____
_____   _____
_____   _____
_____   _____
_____   _____
_____   _____
_____   _____
_____   _____
_____   _____

Notes

_____
_____
_____

Recipe: _____

Serving: _____   Prep Time: _____

Cook Time: _____   Temperature: _____

Ingredients:

_____
_____
_____
_____
_____
_____
_____
_____
_____
_____
_____
_____
_____
_____
_____
_____
_____
_____
_____

Methods:

_____
_____
_____
_____
_____
_____
_____
_____
_____
_____
_____
_____
_____
_____
_____
_____
_____
_____
_____

Notes

_____
_____
_____

Recipe: _____

Serving: _____ Prep Time: _____

Cook Time: _____ Temperature: _____

Ingredients:

_____
_____
_____
_____
_____
_____
_____
_____
_____
_____
_____
_____
_____
_____
_____
_____
_____
_____
_____
_____
_____
_____
_____

Methods:

_____
_____
_____
_____
_____
_____
_____
_____
_____
_____
_____
_____
_____
_____
_____
_____
_____
_____
_____
_____
_____
_____
_____

Notes

_____
_____
_____

Recipe: _____

Serving: _____ Prep Time: _____

Cook Time: _____ Temperature: _____

Ingredients: Methods:
_____   _____
_____   _____
_____   _____
_____   _____
_____   _____
_____   _____
_____   _____
_____   _____
_____   _____
_____   _____
_____   _____
_____   _____
_____   _____
_____   _____
_____   _____
_____   _____
_____   _____

Notes

_____
_____
_____

Recipe: _____

Serving: _____ Prep Time: _____

Cook Time: _____ Temperature: _____

Ingredients:

_____
_____
_____
_____
_____
_____
_____
_____
_____
_____
_____
_____
_____
_____
_____
_____
_____
_____
_____
_____
_____
_____

Methods:

_____
_____
_____
_____
_____
_____
_____
_____
_____
_____
_____
_____
_____
_____
_____
_____
_____
_____
_____
_____
_____
_____

Notes

_____
_____

Recipe: _____

Serving: _____   Prep Time: _____

Cook Time: _____   Temperature: _____

Ingredients: Methods:

_____   _____
_____   _____
_____   _____
_____   _____
_____   _____
_____   _____
_____   _____
_____   _____
_____   _____
_____   _____
_____   _____
_____   _____
_____   _____
_____   _____
_____   _____
_____   _____
_____   _____

Notes

_____
_____
_____

Recipe: _____

Serving: _____   Prep Time: _____

Cook Time: _____   Temperature: _____

Ingredients:

_____
_____
_____
_____
_____
_____
_____
_____
_____
_____
_____
_____
_____
_____
_____
_____
_____
_____

Methods:

_____
_____
_____
_____
_____
_____
_____
_____
_____
_____
_____
_____
_____
_____
_____
_____
_____
_____

Notes

_____
_____
_____

Recipe: _____

Serving: _____   Prep Time: _____

Cook Time: _____   Temperature: _____

Ingredients: Methods:

_____ _____
_____ _____
_____ _____
_____ _____
_____ _____
_____ _____
_____ _____
_____ _____
_____ _____
_____ _____
_____ _____
_____ _____
_____ _____
_____ _____
_____ _____
_____ _____
_____ _____

Notes

_____
_____
_____

Recipe: _____

Serving: _____   Prep Time: _____

Cook Time: _____   Temperature: _____

Ingredients: Methods:

_____   _____
_____   _____
_____   _____
_____   _____
_____   _____
_____   _____
_____   _____
_____   _____
_____   _____
_____   _____
_____   _____
_____   _____
_____   _____
_____   _____
_____   _____
_____   _____
_____   _____

Notes

_____
_____
_____

Recipe: _____

Serving: _____   Prep Time: _____

Cook Time: _____   Temperature: _____

Ingredients:

_____
_____
_____
_____
_____
_____
_____
_____
_____
_____
_____
_____
_____
_____
_____
_____
_____
_____
_____

Methods:

_____
_____
_____
_____
_____
_____
_____
_____
_____
_____
_____
_____
_____
_____
_____
_____
_____
_____
_____

Notes

_____
_____
_____

Recipe: _____

Serving: _____   Prep Time: _____

Cook Time: _____   Temperature: _____

Ingredients:

_____
_____
_____
_____
_____
_____
_____
_____
_____
_____
_____
_____
_____
_____
_____
_____
_____
_____

Methods:

_____
_____
_____
_____
_____
_____
_____
_____
_____
_____
_____
_____
_____
_____
_____
_____
_____
_____

Notes

_____
_____
_____

Recipe: _____

Serving: _____ **Prep Time:** _____

Cook Time: _____ **Temperature:** _____

Ingredients:

_____
_____
_____
_____
_____
_____
_____
_____
_____
_____
_____
_____
_____
_____
_____
_____
_____

Methods:

_____
_____
_____
_____
_____
_____
_____
_____
_____
_____
_____
_____
_____
_____
_____
_____
_____

Notes

_____
_____
_____

Recipe: _____

Serving: _____   Prep Time: _____

Cook Time: _____ Temperature: _____

Ingredients: Methods:

Notes

Recipe: _____

Serving: _____   Prep Time: _____

Cook Time: _____   Temperature: _____

Ingredients: Methods:
_____   _____
_____   _____
_____   _____
_____   _____
_____   _____
_____   _____
_____   _____
_____   _____
_____   _____
_____   _____
_____   _____
_____   _____
_____   _____
_____   _____
_____   _____
_____   _____
_____   _____
_____   _____

Notes

_____
_____
_____

Recipe: _____

Serving: _____ Prep Time: _____

Cook Time: _____ Temperature: _____

Ingredients: Methods:

_____   _____
_____   _____
_____   _____
_____   _____
_____   _____
_____   _____
_____   _____
_____   _____
_____   _____
_____   _____
_____   _____
_____   _____
_____   _____
_____   _____
_____   _____
_____   _____

Notes

_____
_____
_____

Recipe: _____

Serving: _____   Prep Time: _____

Cook Time: _____ Temperature: _____

Ingredients:

_____
_____
_____
_____
_____
_____
_____
_____
_____
_____
_____
_____
_____
_____
_____
_____
_____

Methods:

_____
_____
_____
_____
_____
_____
_____
_____
_____
_____
_____
_____
_____
_____
_____
_____
_____

Notes

_____
_____
_____

Recipe: _____

Serving: _____   Prep Time: _____

Cook Time: _____   Temperature: _____

Ingredients:

_____
_____
_____
_____
_____
_____
_____
_____
_____
_____
_____
_____
_____
_____
_____
_____
_____
_____

Methods:

_____
_____
_____
_____
_____
_____
_____
_____
_____
_____
_____
_____
_____
_____
_____
_____
_____
_____

Notes

_____
_____
_____

Recipe: _____

Serving: _____ Prep Time: _____

Cook Time: _____ Temperature: _____

Ingredients:

_____
_____
_____
_____
_____
_____
_____
_____
_____
_____
_____
_____
_____
_____
_____
_____
_____
_____
_____
_____
_____

Methods:

_____
_____
_____
_____
_____
_____
_____
_____
_____
_____
_____
_____
_____
_____
_____
_____
_____
_____
_____
_____
_____

Notes

_____
_____
_____

Recipe: _____

Serving: _____ Prep Time: _____

Cook Time: _____ Temperature: _____

Ingredients:

Methods:

Notes

www.ingramcontent.com/pod-product-compliance
Lightning Source LLC
Chambersburg PA
CBHW080545220526
45466CB00010B/3039